NURSING
Crossword Puzzle for student nurses
Volume 1
Issue 1

PHARMACOLOGY

Evelyn Justiniano LPN, GRN

ANTICONVULSANTS MEDICATIONS

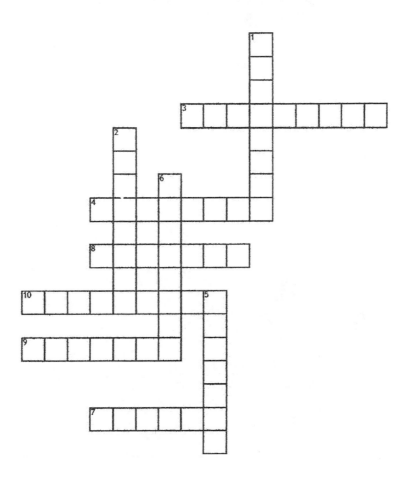

Across

3. What is Gabapentin trade name?
4. What is Lamotrigine trade name?
7. What is Pregabalin trade name?
8. What is Topiramate trade name?
9. What is Valproate trade name?
10. What is Oxcarbazepine trade name?

Down

1. What is Carbamazepine trade name?
2. What is Divaproex Sodium trade name?
5. What is Phenobarbital trade name?
6. What is phenytoin trade name?

ANTIPLATELET, ANTICOAGULANT, THROMBOLYTIC MEDICATIONS

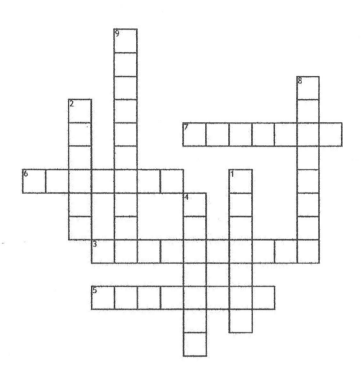

Across

3. What is dipyridamole trade name?
5. What is warfarin trade name?
6. What is enoxaparin trade name?
7. What is rivaroxaban trade Name?

Down

1. What is aspirin trade name?
2. What is clopidogrel trade name?
4. What is dabigatran etexilate trade name?
8. What is alteplase trade name?
9. What is urokinase trade name?

CARDIOVASCULAR MEDICATIONS

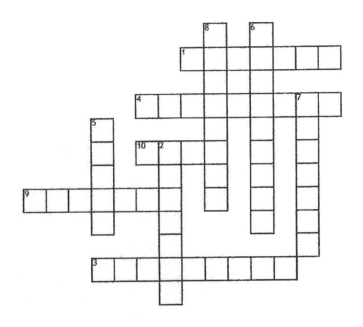

Across

1. What is Captopril's trade name?
3. What is Nitroglycerin's trade name?
4. What is Amiodarone's trade name?
9. What is Atorvastatin's trade name?
10. What is Hydrochlorothiazide's trade name?

Down

2. What is Doxazosin Mesylate's trade name?
5. What is Furosemide's trade name?
6. What is Metoprolol Tartrate's trade name?
7. What is amlodipine Besylate's trade name?
8. What is Diltiazem's trade name?

DIABETIC MEDICATIONS

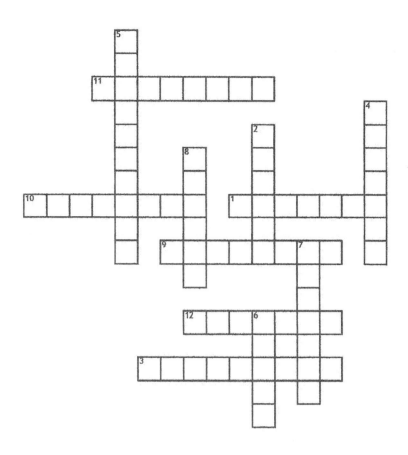

Across

1. What is Acarbose trade name?

3. What is Glipizide trade name?

9. What is Insulin Regular trade name?

10. What is Glucagon trade name?

11. What is Insulin Isophane suspection trade name?

12. What is Insulin Lispro trade name?

Down

2. What is Glimepiride trade name?

4. What is Glyburide trade name?

5. What is Metformin HCL trade name?

6. What is pioglitazone HCL trade name?

7. What is Insulin Aspart trade name?

8. What is Insuline Glargine trade name?

ALLERGY & ASTHMA, ANALGESICS, ANTINEOPLASTICS MEDICATIONS

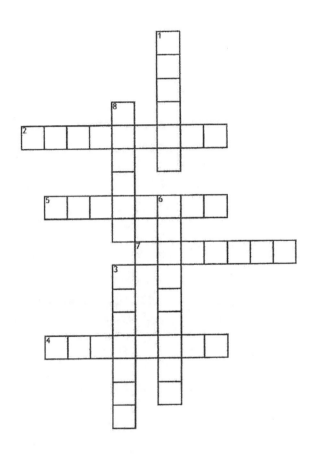

Across

2. What is Beclomethasone trade name?

4. What is Celecoxib trade name?

5. What is Hydromorphone trade name?

7. What is Methotrexate trade name?

Down

1. What is Certizine HCL trade name?

3. What is Acetaminophen trade name?

6. What is Morphine trade name?

8. What is Hydrocodone Acetaminophen trade name?

SEIZURE MEDICATIONS

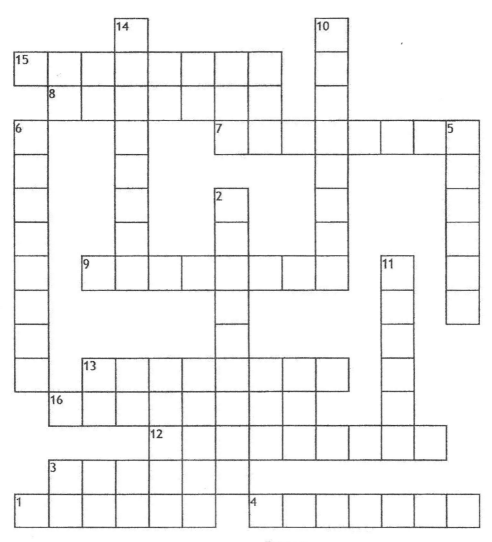

Across

1. What is diazepam trade name?
3. What is lorazepam trade name?
4. What is phenobarbital trade name?
7. What is tiagabine trade name?
8. What is topiramate trade name?
9. What is carbamazepine trade name?
12. What is oxcarbazepine trade name?
13. What is phenytoin trade name?
15. What is zonisamide trade name?
16. What is ethosuximide trade name?

Down

2. What is gabapentin trade name?
5. What is pregabalin trade name?
6. What is primidone trade name?
10. What is Lamotrigine trade name?
11. What is levitiracetam trade name?
14. What is valproic acid trade name?

PAIN MANAGEMENT OPIOID MEDICATIONS

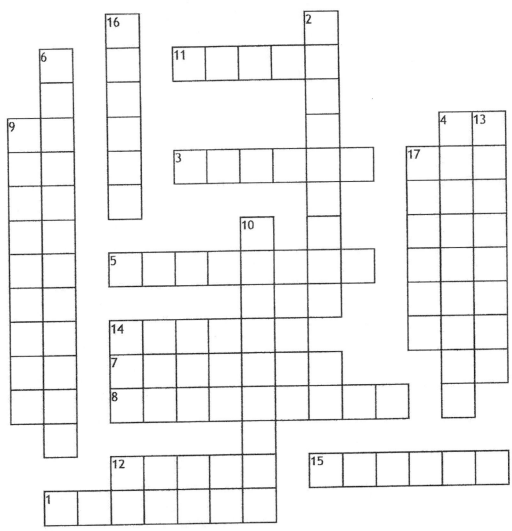

Across

1. What is Hydrocodone bitartrate trade name?

3. What is Propoxyphene HCL trade name?

5. What is Hydromorphone HCL trade name?

7. What is Meperidine trade name?

8. What is Methadone hydrochloride trade name?

11. What is Nalmefene hydrochloride trade name?

12. What is Naltrexone hydrochloride trade name?

14. What is Butorphanol tartrate trade name?

15. What is Dezocine trade name?

Down

2. What is Oxycodone HCL trade name?

4. What is Fentanyl trade name?

6. What is Levorphanol tartrate trade name?

9. What is Morphine sulfate trade name?

10. What is Oxymorphone hydrochloride?

13. What is Buprenorpine hydrochloride trade name?

16. What is Nalbuphine hydrocloride trade name?

17. What is Pentazocine hydrocloride trade name?

NON-OPIOID ANALGESIC MEDICATIONS

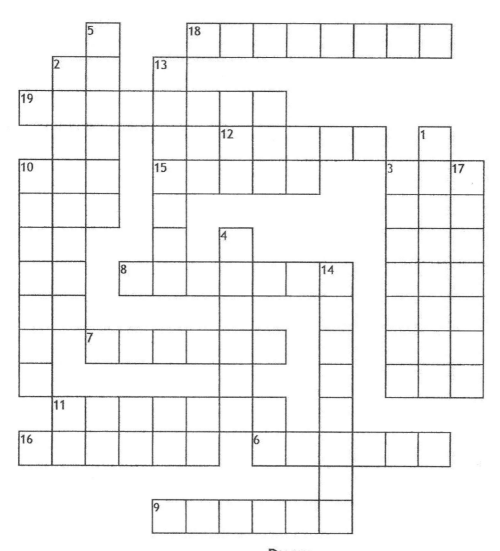

Across

6. What is Flurbiprofen trade name?
7. What is Ibuprofen trade name?
8. What is Indomethacin trade name?
9. What is Ketoprofen trade name?
11. What is Mefenamic acid trade name?
12. What is Meloxicam trade name?
15. What is Naproxen sodium trade name?
16. What is Oxaprozin trad name?
18. What is Sulindac trade name?
19. What is tolmetin trade name?

Down

1. What is Celecoxib trade name?
2. What is Diclofenac trade name?
3. What is Diflunisal trade name?
4. What is Etodolac trade name?
5. What is Fenoprofen calcium trade name?
10. What is Ketorolac tromethamine trade name?
13. What is Nabumetone trade name?
14. What is Naproxen trade name?
17. What is Piroxicam trade name?

TERMINATING & PREVENTING ANTI-MIGRAINE MEDICATIONS

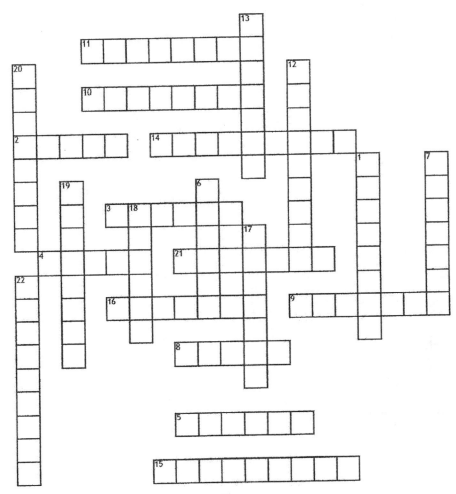

Across

2. What is almotriptan trade name?
3. What is eletriptan trade name?
4. What is frovatriptan trade name?
5. What is naratriptan trade name?
8. What is zolmitriptan trade name?
9. What is topiramate trade name?
10. What is valproic acid trade name?
11. What is atenolol trade name?
14. What is timolol trade name?
15. What is nifedipine trade name?
16. What is nimodipine trade name?
21. What is methysergide trade name?

Down

1. What is ergotamine tartrate trade name?
6. What is ritatriptan trade name?
7. What is sumatriptan trade name?
12. What is metoprolol trade name?
13. What is propranolol trade name?
17. What is verapamil trade name?
18. What is Amitriptyline HCL trade name?
19. What is imipramine trade name?
20. What is Protriptyline trade name?
22. What is riboflavin trade name?

BENZODIAZEPINES FOR ANXIETY & INSOMNIA MEDICATIONS

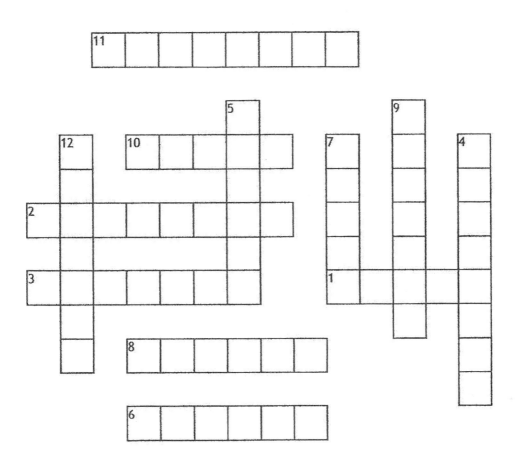

Across

1. What is Alprazolam trade name?
2. What is Clonazepam trade name?
3. What is Chlordiazepoxide trade name?
6. What is Lorazepam trade name?
8. What is Estazolam trade name?
10. What is Quazepam trade name?
11. What is Temazepam trade name?

Down

4. What is Clorazepate trade name?
5. What is Diazepam trade name?
7. What is Oxazepam trade name?
9. What is Flurazepam trade name?
12. What is Triazolam trade name?

RESPIRATORY MEDICATIONS I

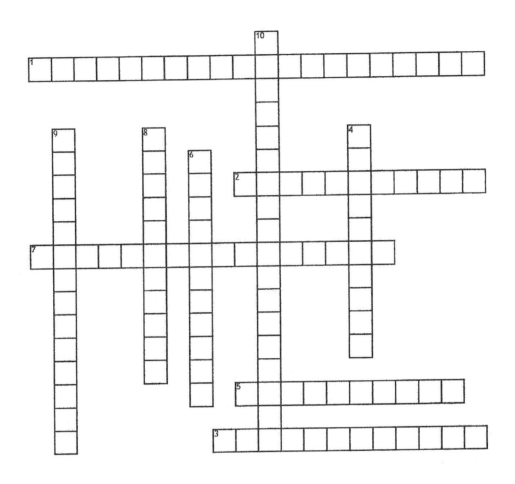

Across
1. What is Combivent's generic name?
2. What is Singulair's generic name?
3. What is Theo Dur generic name?
5. What is Spiriva's generic name?
7. What is ProAir's generic name?

Down
4. What is Serevent's generic name?
6. What is Tessalon generic name?
8. What is Robitussin's generic name?
9. What is NasalCom's generic name?
10. What is Atrovent's generic name?

RESPIRATORY MEDICATIONS II

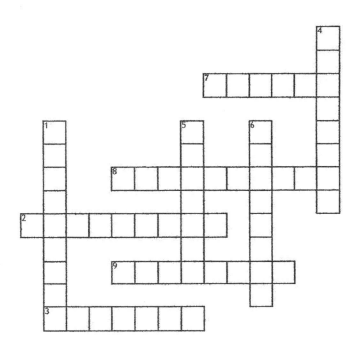

Across
2. What is Montelukast's trade name?
3. What is Theophylline's trade name?
7. What is Albuterol sulfate' trade name?
8. What is Guaifenesin's trade name?
9. What is Cromolyn sodium's trade name?

Down
1. What is Albuterol/Ipratropium's trade name?
4. What is Salmeterol trade name?
5. What is Tiotropium's trade name?
6. What is Benzonatate's trade name?

CARDIOVASCULAR MEDICATIONS

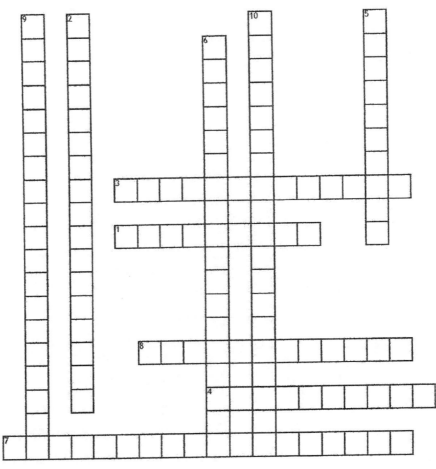

Across

1. What is Capoten's generic name?
3. What is Nitrostat's generic name?
4. What is Cardarone generic name?
7. What is Norvasc's generic name?
8. What is Cardizem's generic name?

Down

2. What is Cardura's generic name?
5. What is Lasix's generic name?
6. What is Lopressor's generic name?
9. What is Lipitor's generic name?
10. What is HCTZ generic name?

ANTIPLATELET, ANTICOAGULANT, THROMBOLYTIC MEDICATIONS

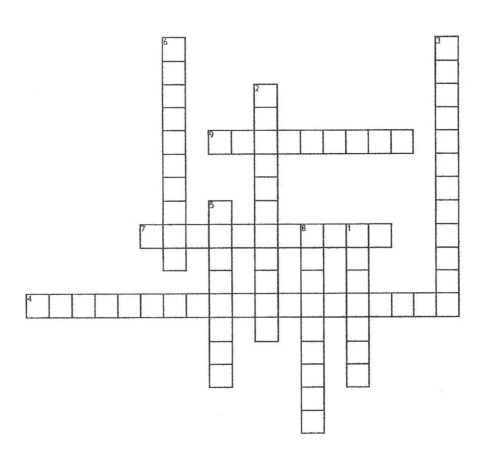

Across

4. What is Pradaxa generic name?
7. What is Xarelto generic name?
9. What is Abbokinase generic name?

Down

1. What is of Ecotrin generic name?
2. What is Plavix generic name?
3. What is Persantine generic name?
5. What is Coumadin generic Name?
6. What is Lovenox generic name?
8. What is Activase generic name?

ANTI-INFECTIVES MEDICATIONS I

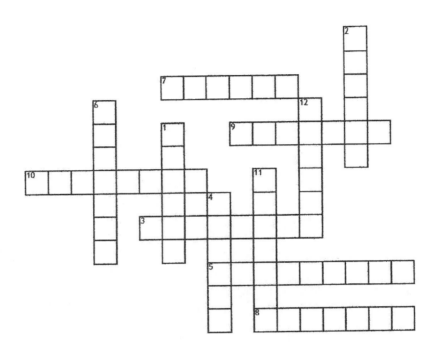

Across

3. What is Fluconazole's trade name?
5. What is Gentamycin's trade name?
7. What is Cephalexin's trade name?
8. What is Amoxicillin's trade name?
9. What is ampicillin's trade name?
10. What is penicillin's trade name?

Down

1. What is Amikin's trade name?
2. What is Tobramycin's trade name?
4. What is Metronidazole's trade name?
6. What is Oseltamivir Phosphate's trade name?
11. What is trimethoprim sulfamethoxazole trade name?
12. What is Clarithromycin trade name?

ANTI-INFECTIVES MEDICATION II

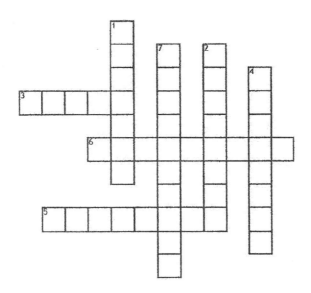

Across

3. What is ciprofloxacin's trade name?
5. What is vancomycin's trade name?
6. What is azithromycin's trade name?

Down

1. What is cefoxitin's trade name?
2. What is cefotaxime trade name?
4. What is levofloxacin's trade name?
7. What is erythromycin' trade name?

ANTI-INFECTIVES MEDICATIONS III

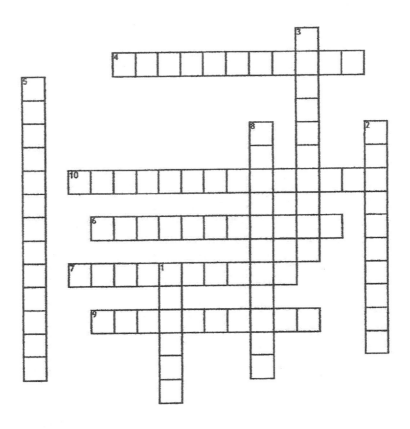

Across
4. What is Diflucan's generic name?
6. What is Tamiflu's generic name?
7. What is Keflex's generic name?
9. What is Bicillin's trade name?
10. What is Biaxin trade name?

Down
1. What is Amikin's generic name?
2. What is Garamycin's generic name?
3. What is Tobrex generic name?
5. What is flagyl's generic name?
8. What is Motag's generic name?

ANTI-INFECTIVES MEDICATIONS IV

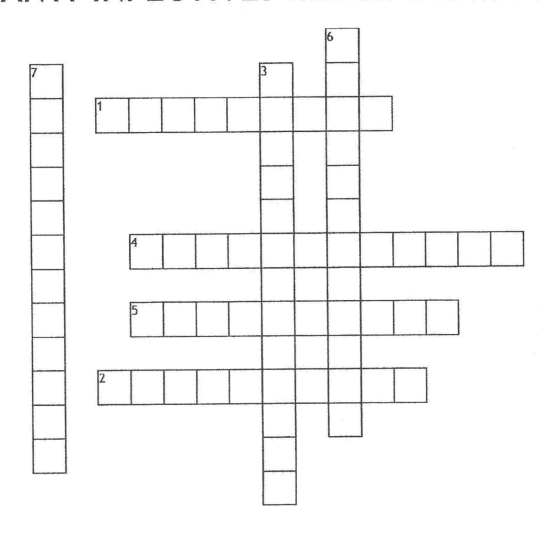

Across

1. What is Mefoxin's generic name?
2. What is Clarforan generic name?
4. What is Levaquin's generic name?
5. What is Vancocin's generic name?

Down

3. What is Cipro's generic name?
6. What is Zithromax's generic name?
7. What is Erytrocin's generic name?

DIABETIC MEDICATIONS

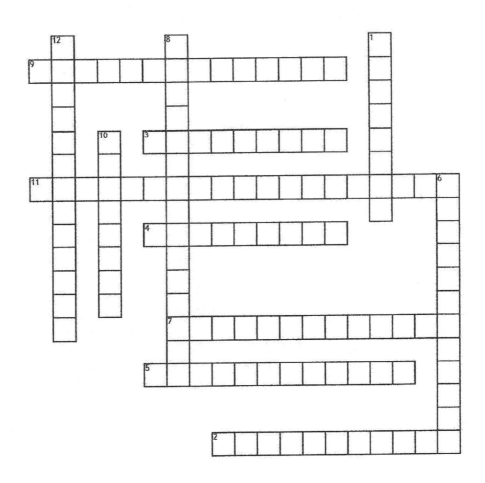

Across

2. What is Amaryl generic name?
3. What is Glucotrol generic name?
4. What is DiaBeta generic name?
5. What is Glucophage generic name?
7. What is NovoLog generic name?
9. What is Humulin R generic name?
11. What is Humulin N generic name?

Down

1. What is Precose generic name?
6. What is Actos generic name?
8. What is Lantus trade name?
10. What is GlucaGen generic name?
12. What is Humalog generic name?

ALLERGY & ASTHMA, ANALGESICS, ANTINEOPLASTIC MEDICATIONS

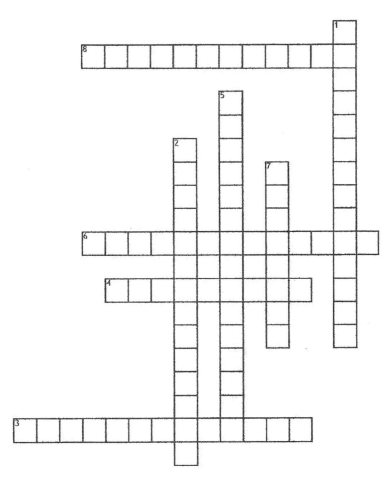

Across

3. What is Tylenol generic name?
4. What is Celebrex generic name?
6. What is Dilaudid generic name?
8. What is Trexall generic name?

Down

1. What is Zyrtec generic name?
2. What is Beclovent generic name?
5. What is Lortab generic name?
7. What is Duramorph generic name?

TRICYLIC ANTIDEPRESSANTS (TCAs) & MONOAMINE OXIDASE INHIBITORS (MAOIs) & ATYPICAL ANTIDEPRESSANT

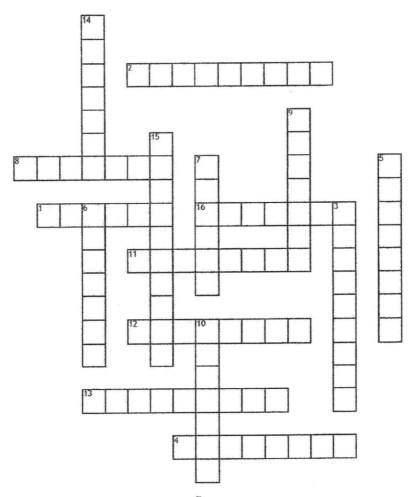

Across

1. What is Amitriptyline trade name?
2. What is Clomipramine trade name?
4. What is Doxepin trade name?
8. What is Tranylcypromine trade name?
11. What s Maprotiline trade name?
12. What is Protriptyline trade name?
13. What is Trimipramine trade name?
16. What is Mirtazapine trade name?

Down

3. What is Desipramine trade name?
5. What is Imipramine trade name?
6. What is Nortriptyline trade name?
7. What is Phenelzine trade name?
9. What is Trazodone trade name?
10. What is Amoxapine trade name?
14. What is Isocarboxazid trade name?
15. What is Bupropion trade name?

PHENOTHIAZINES & PHENOTHIAZINE CONVENTIONAL ANTIPSYCHOTICS & ADVERSE EFFECTS

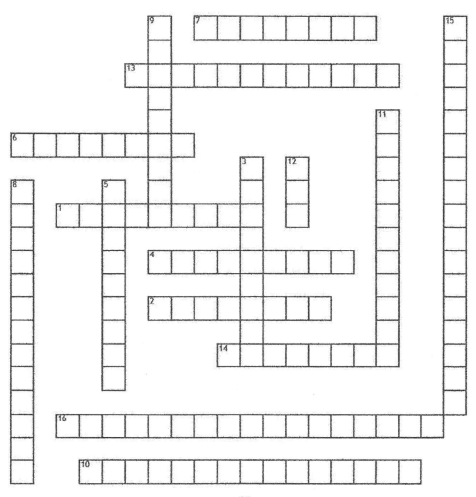

Across

1. What is Chlorpromazine trade name?
2. What is Fluphenazine trade name?
4. What is Prochlorperazine trade name?
6. What is Thioridazine trade name?
7. What is Trifluoperazine trade name?
10. What is effect occurs with dry mouth, tachycardia and blurred vision?
13. Tremors, muscle rigidity, stooped posture, and shuffling gait oscuras with what disease process
14. What is a state of calm or sleep known as?
16. What is known as having odd or strange tongue and face movements with lip smacking?

Down

3. What is Perphenazine trade name?
5. What is Thioridazine trade name?
8. What consist of severe spasms of the back, tongue and facial muscles with twitching movements?
9. What describes constant pacing with repetitive compulsive movements?
11. What can occur when moving quickly to stand from a sitting position?
12. What disorder can occur with having high fever, confusion, muscle ridgity, and elevated serum CK level and can be deadly?
15. When you are impotence and have a diminished libido this is known as having a

HEART FAILURE MEDICATIONS

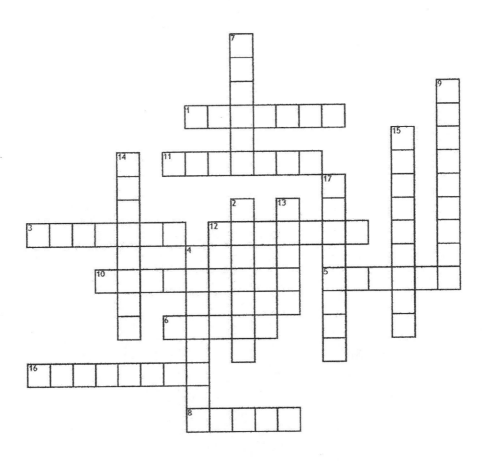

Across

1. What is captopril trade name?
3. What is lisinopril trade name?
5. What is ramipril trade name?
6. What is bumetanide trade name?
8. What is furosemide trade name?
10. What is spironolactone trade name?
11. What is torsemide trade name?
12. What is digoxin trade name?
16. What is nesiritide trade name?

Down

2. What is enalapril trade name?
4. What is quinapril trade name?
7. What is eplerenone trade name?
9. What is Hydrochlorothiazide trade name?
13. What is carvedilol trade name?
14. What is metoprolol Succinate trade name?
15. What is hydralazine with isosorbide trade name?
17. What is inamrinone trade name?

SODIUM, POTASSIUM & CALCIUM CHANNEL BLOCKERS

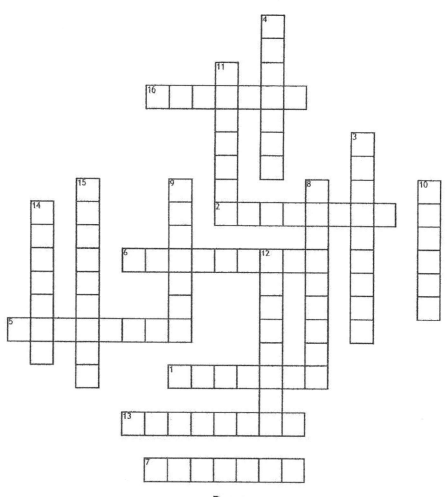

Across
1. What is disopyramide trade name?
2. What is flecainide trade name?
5. What is phenytoin trade name?
6. What is procainamide trade name?
7. What is propafenone trade name?
13. What is diltiazem trade name?
16. What is digoxin trade name?

Down
3. What is lidocaine trade name?
4. What is mexiletine trade name?
8. What is amiodarone trade name?
9. What is dofetilide trade name?
10. What is dronedarone trade name?
11. What is ibutilide trade name?
12. What is sotalol trade name?
14. What is verapamil trade name?
15. What is adenosine trade name?

ANTICONVULSANTS MEDICATIONS

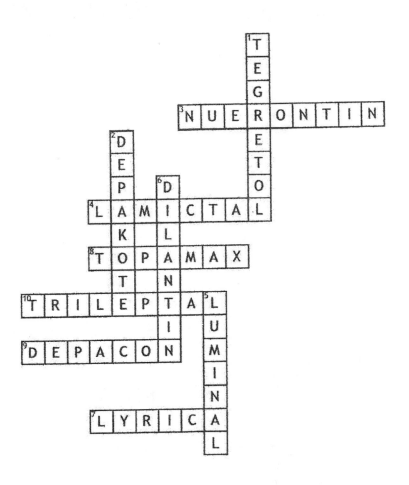

Across

3. What is Gabapentin trade name?
4. What is Lamotrigine trade name?
7. What is Pregabalin trade name?
8. What is Topiramate trade name?
9. What is Valproate trade name?
10. What is Oxcarbazepine trade name?

Down

1. What is Carbamazepine trade name?
2. What is Divaproex Sodium trade name?
5. What is Phenobarbital trade name?
6. What is phenytoin trade name?

ANTIPLATELET, ANTICOAGULANT, THROMBOLYTIC MEDICATIONS

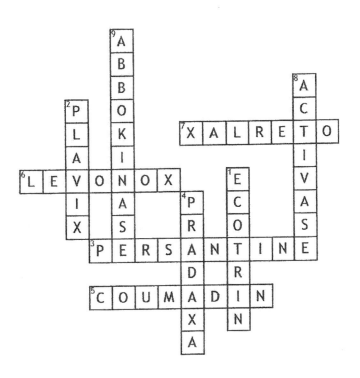

Across

3. What is dipyridamole trade name?
5. What is warfarin trade name?
6. What is enoxaparin trade name?
7. What is rivaroxaban trade Name?

Down

1. What is aspirin trade name?
2. What is clopidogrel trade name?
4. What is dabigatran etexilate trade name?
8. What is alteplase trade name?
9. What is urokinase trade name?

CARDIOVASCULAR MEDICATIONS

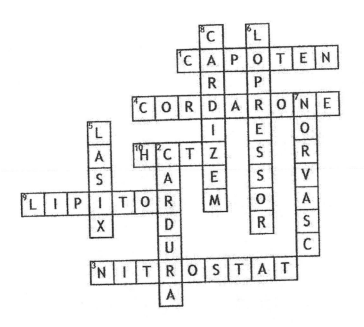

Across

1. What is Captopril's trade name?
3. What is Nitroglycerin's trade name?
4. What is Amiodarone's trade name?
9. What is Atorvastatin's trade name?
10. What is Hydrochlorothiazide's trade name?

Down

2. What is Doxazosin Mesylate's trade name?
5. What is Furosemide's trade name?
6. What is Metoprolol Tartrate's trade name?
7. What is amlodipine Besylate's trade name?
8. What is Diltiazem's trade name?

DIABETIC MEDICATIONS

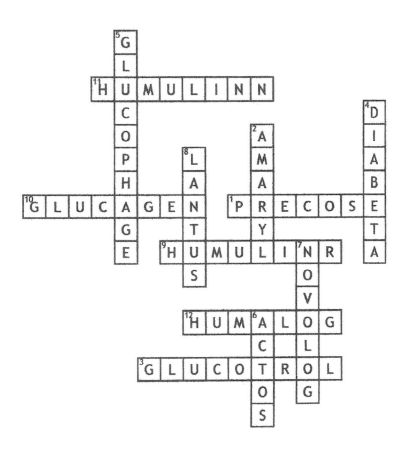

Across
1. What is Acarbose trade name?
3. What is Glipizide trade name?
9. What is Insulin Regular trade name?
10. What is Glucagon trade name?
11. What is Insulin Isophane suspection trade name?
12. What is Insulin Lispro trade name?

Down
2. What is Glimepiride trade name?
4. What is Glyburide trade name?
5. What is Metformin HCL trade name?
6. What is pioglitazone HCL trade name?
7. What is Insulin Aspart trade name?
8. What is Insuline Glargine trade name?

ALLERGY & ASTHMA, ANALGESICS, ANTINEOPLASTICS MEDICATIONS

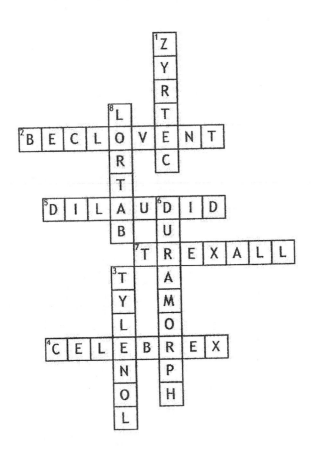

Across

2. What is Beclomethasone trade name?
4. What is Celecoxib trade name?
5. What is Hydromorphone trade name?
7. What is Methotrexate trade name?

Down

1. What is Certizine HCL trade name?
3. What is Acetaminophen trade name?
6. What is Morphine trade name?
8. What is Hydrocodone Acetaminophen trade name?

SEIZURE MEDICATIONS

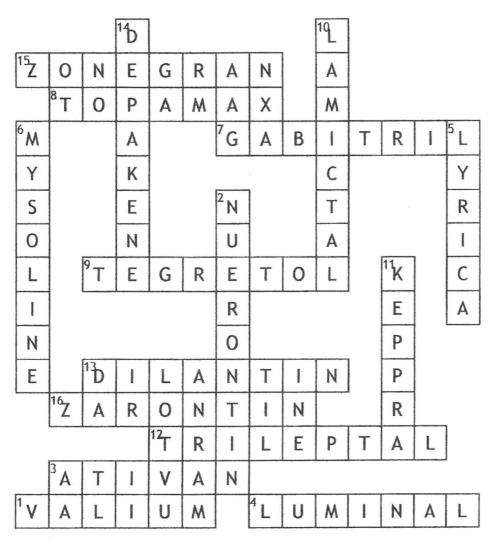

Across
1. What is diazepam trade name?
3. What is lorazepam trade name?
4. What is phenobarbital trade name?
7. What is tiagabine trade name?
8. What is topiramate trade name?
9. What is carbamazepine trade name?
12. What is oxcarbazepine trade name?
13. What is phenytoin trade name?
15. What is zonisamide trade name?
16. What is ethosuximide trade name?

Down
2. What is gabapentin trade name?
5. What is pregabalin trade name?
6. What is primidone trade name?
10. What is Lamotrigine trade name?
11. What is levitiracetam trade name?
14. What is valproic acid trade name?

PAIN MANAGEMENT OPIOID MEDICATIONS

Across
1. What is Hydrocodone bitartrate trade name?
3. What is Propoxyphene HCL trade name?
5. What is Hydromorphone HCL trade name?
7. What is Meperidine trade name?
8. What is Methadone hydrochloride trade name?
11. What is Nalmefene hydrochloride trade name?
12. What is Naltrexone hydrochloride trade name?
14. What is Butorphanol tartrate trade name?
15. What is Dezocine trade name?

Down
2. What is Oxycodone HCL trade name?
4. What is Fentanyl trade name?
6. What is Levorphanol tartrate trade name?
9. What is Morphine sulfate trade name?
10. What is Oxymorphone hydrochloride?
13. What is Buprenorpine hydrochloride trade name?
16. What is Nalbuphine hydrocloride trade name?
17. What is Pentazocine hydrocloride trade name?

NON-OPIOID ANALGESIC MEDICATIONS

Across

6. What is Flurbiprofen trade name?
7. What is Ibuprofen trade name?
8. What is Indomethacin trade name?
9. What is Ketoprofen trade name?
11. What is Mefenamic acid trade name?
12. What is Meloxicam trade name?
15. What is Naproxen sodium trade name?
16. What is Oxaprozin trad name?
18. What is Sulindac trade name?
19. What is tolmetin trade name?

Down

1. What is Celecoxib trade name?
2. What is Diclofenac trade name?
3. What is Diflunisal trade name?
4. What is Etodolac trade name?
5. What is Fenoprofen calcium trade name?
10. What is Ketorolac tromethamine trade name?
13. What is Nabumetone trade name?
14. What is Naproxen trade name?
17. What is Piroxicam trade name?

TERMINATING & PREVENTING ANTI-MIGRAINE MEDICATIONS

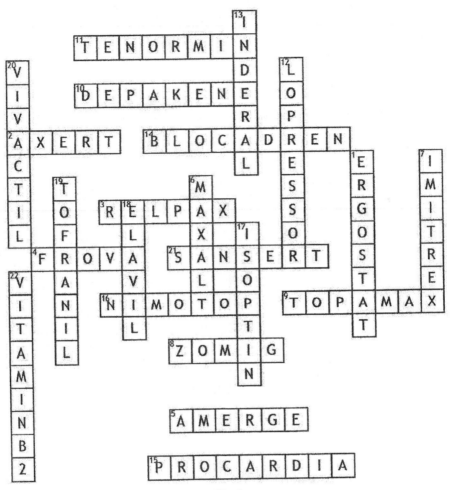

Across

2. What is almotriptan trade name?
3. What is eletriptan trade name?
4. What is frovatriptan trade name?
5. What is naratriptan trade name?
8. What is zolmitriptan trade name?
9. What is topiramate trade name?
10. What is valproic acid trade name?
11. What is atenolol trade name?
14. What is timolol trade name?
15. What is nifedipine trade name?
16. What is nimodipine trade name?
21. What is methysergide trade name?

Down

1. What is ergotamine tartrate trade name?
6. What is ritatriptan trade name?
7. What is sumatriptan trade name?
12. What is metoprolol trade name?
13. What is propranolol trade name?
17. What is verapamil trade name?
18. What is Amitriptyline HCL trade name?
19. What is imipramine trade name?
20. What is Protriptyline trade name?
22. What is riboflavin trade name?

BENZODIAZEPINES FOR ANXIETY & INSOMNIA MEDICATIONS

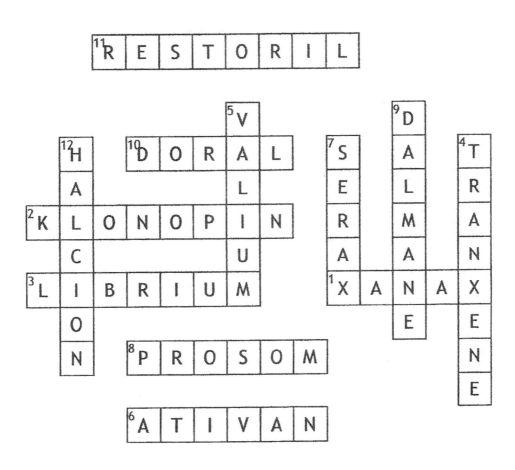

Across
1. What is Alprazolam trade name?
2. What is Clonazepam trade name?
3. What is Chlordiazepoxide trade name?
6. What is Lorazepam trade name?
8. What is Estazolam trade name?
10. What is Quazepam trade name?
11. What is Temazepam trade name?

Down
4. What is Clorazepate trade name?
5. What is Diazepam trade name?
7. What is Oxazepam trade name?
9. What is Flurazepam trade name?
12. What is Triazolam trade name?

RESPIRATORY MEDICATIONS I

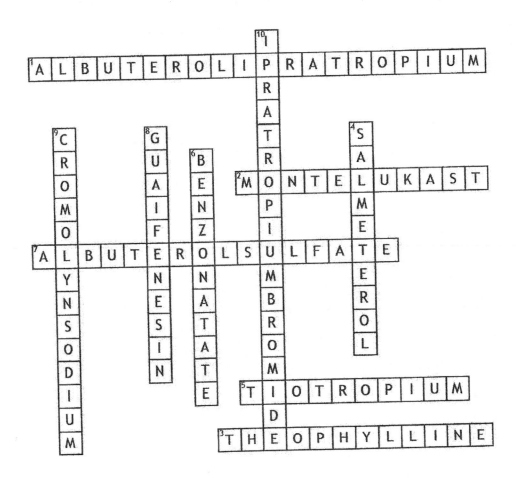

Across
1. What is Combivent's generic name?
2. What is Singulair's generic name?
3. What is Theo Dur generic name?
5. What is Spiriva's generic name?
7. What is ProAir's generic name?

Down
4. What is Serevent's generic name?
6. What is Tessalon generic name?
8. What is Robitussin's generic name?
9. What is NasalCom's generic name?
10. What is Atrovent's generic name?

RESPIRATORY MEDICATIONS II

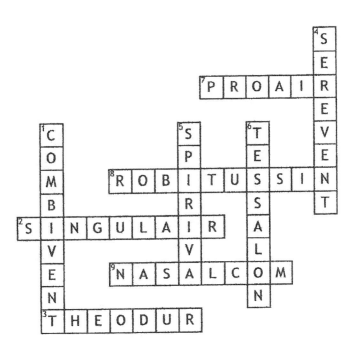

Across

2. What is Montelukast's trade name?
3. What is Theophylline's trade name?
7. What is Albuterol sulfate' trade name?
8. What is Guaifenesin's trade name?
9. What is Cromolyn sodium's trade name?

Down

1. What is Albuterol/Ipratropium's trade name?
4. What is Salmeterol trade name?
5. What is Tiotropium's trade name?
6. What is Benzonatate's trade name?

CARDIOVASCULAR MEDICATIONS

Down (9): ATORVASTATINCALCIUM

Down (2): DOXAZOSINMESYLATE

Down (6): METOPROLOLTARTRATE

Down (10): HYDROCHLOROTHIAZIDE

Down (5): FUROSEMIDE

Across (3): NITROGLYCERIN

Across (1): CAPTOPRIL

Across (8): DILTIAZEMHCL

Across (4): AMIODARONE

Across (7): AMLODIPINEBESYLATE

Across

1. What is Capoten's generic name?
3. What is Nitrostat's generic name?
4. What is Cardarone generic name?
7. What is Norvasc's generic name?
8. What is Cardizem's generic name?

Down

2. What is Cardura's generic name?
5. What is Lasix's generic name?
6. What is Lopressor's generic name?
9. What is Lipitor's generic name?
10. What is HCTZ generic name?

ANTIPLATELET, ANTICOAGULANT, THROMBOLYTIC MEDICATIONS

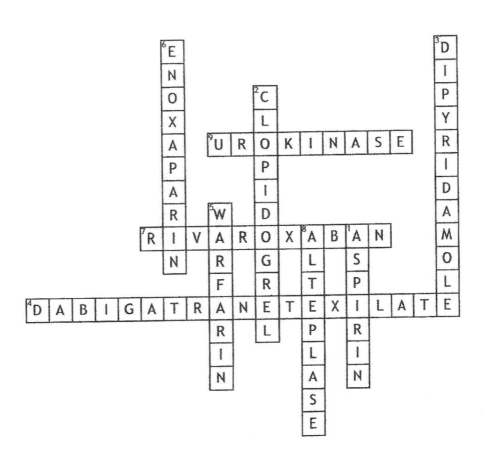

Across

4. What is Pradaxa generic name?
7. What is Xarelto generic name?
9. What is Abbokinase generic name?

Down

1. What is of Ecotrin generic name?
2. What is Plavix generic name?
3. What is Persantine generic name?
5. What is Coumadin generic Name?
6. What is Lovenox generic name?
8. What is Activase generic name?

ANTI-INFECTIVES MEDICATIONS I

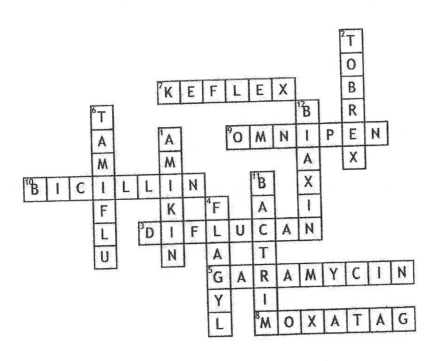

Across

3. What is Fluconazole's trade name?
5. What is Gentamycin's trade name?
7. What is Cephalexin's trade name?
8. What is Amoxicillin's trade name?
9. What is ampicillin's trade name?
10. What is penicillin's trade name?

Down

1. What is Amikin's trade name?
2. What is Tobramycin's trade name?
4. What is Metronidazole's trade name?
6. What is Oseltamivir Phosphate's trade name?
11. What is trimethoprim sulfamethoxazole trade name?
12. What is Clarithromycin trade name?

ANTI-INFECTIVES MEDICATION II

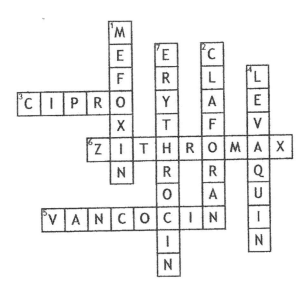

Across

3. What is ciprofloxacin's trade name?
5. What is vancomycin's trade name?
6. What is azithromycin's trade name?

Down

1. What is cefoxitin's trade name?
2. What is cefotaxime trade name?
4. What is levofloxacin's trade name?
7. What is erythromycin' trade name?

ANTI-INFECTIVES MEDICATIONS III

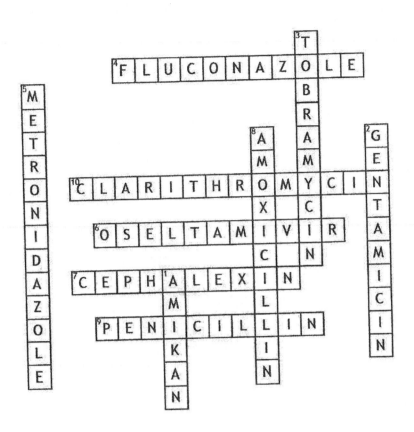

Across
4. What is Diflucan's generic name?
6. What is Tamiflu's generic name?
7. What is Keflex's generic name?
9. What is Bicillin's trade name?
10. What is Biaxin trade name?

Down
1. What is Amikin's generic name?
2. What is Garamycin's generic name?
3. What is Tobrex generic name?
5. What is flagyl's generic name?
8. What is Motag's generic name?

ANTI-INFECTIVES MEDICATIONS IV

```
                                    6A
 7E                        3C        Z
 R    1C  E  F  O  X  I  T  I        N
 Y                         P         T
 T                         R         H
 H                         O         R
 R    4L  E  V  O  F  L  O  X  A  C  I  N
 O                         L         M
 M    5V  A  N  C  O  M  Y  C  I  N
 Y                         X         C
 C    2C  E  F  O  T  A  X  I  M  E
 I                         C         N
 N                         I
                           N
```

Across

1. What is Mefoxin's generic name?
2. What is Clarforan generic name?
4. What is Levaquin's generic name?
5. What is Vancocin's generic name?

Down

3. What is Cipro's generic name?
6. What is Zithromax's generic name?
7. What is Erytrocin's generic name?

DIABETIC MEDICATIONS

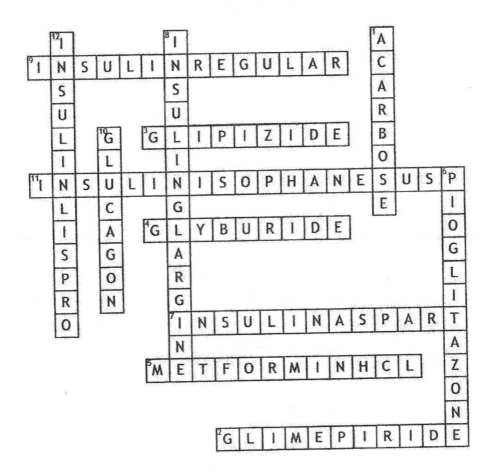

Across

2. What is Amaryl generic name?
3. What is Glucotrol generic name?
4. What is DiaBeta generic name?
5. What is Glucophage generic name?
7. What is NovoLog generic name?
9. What is Humulin R generic name?
11. What is Humulin N generic name?

Down

1. What is Precose generic name?
6. What is Actos generic name?
8. What is Lantus trade name?
10. What is GlucaGen generic name?
12. What is Humalog generic name?

ALLERGY & ASTHMA, ANALGESICS, ANTINEOPLASTIC MEDICATIONS

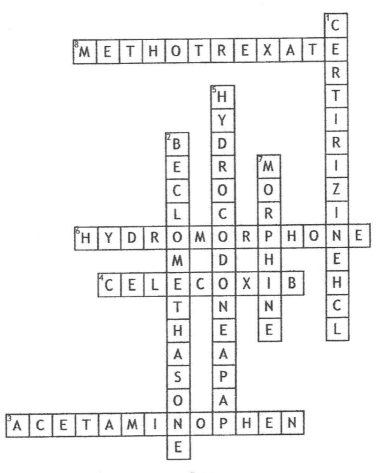

Across

3. What is Tylenol generic name?
4. What is Celebrex generic name?
6. What is Dilaudid generic name?
8. What is Trexall generic name?

Down

1. What is Zyrtec generic name?
2. What is Beclovent generic name?
5. What is Lortab generic name?
7. What is Duramorph generic name?

TRICYLIC ANTIDEPRESSANTS (TCAs) & MONOAMINE OXIDASE INHIBITORS (MAOIs) & ATYPICAL ANTIDEPRESSANT

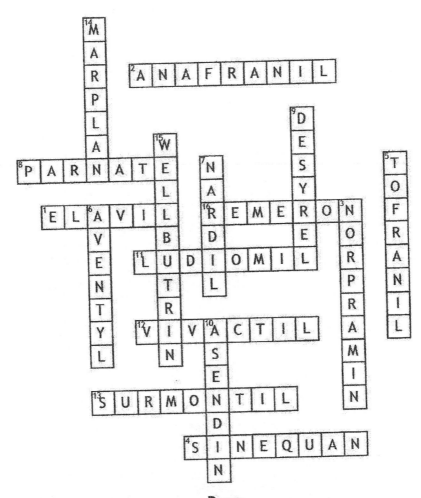

Across

1. What is Amitriptyline trade name?
2. What is Clomipramine trade name?
4. What is Doxepin trade name?
8. What is Tranylcypromine trade name?
11. What s Maprotiline trade name?
12. What is Protriptyline trade name?
13. What is Trimipramine trade name?
16. What is Mirtazapine trade name?

Down

3. What is Desipramine trade name?
5. What is Imipramine trade name?
6. What is Nortriptyline trade name?
7. What is Phenelzine trade name?
9. What is Trazodone trade name?
10. What is Amoxapine trade name?
14. What is Isocarboxazid trade name?
15. What is Bupropion trade name?

PHENOTHIAZINES & PHENOTHIAZINE CONVENTIONAL ANTIPSYCHOTICS & ADVERSE EFFECTS

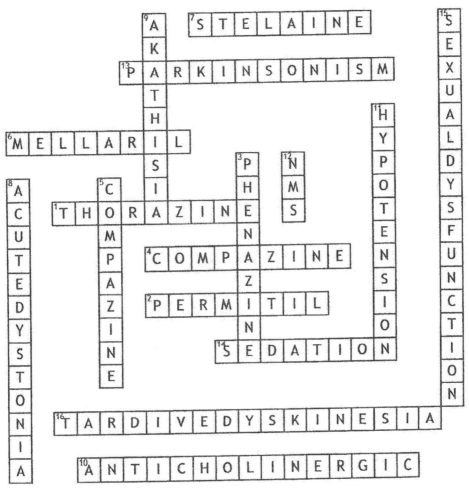

Across

1. What is Chlorpromazine trade name?
2. What is Fluphenazine trade name?
4. What is Prochlorperazine trade name?
6. What is Thioridazine trade name?
7. What is Trifluoperazine trade name?
10. What is effect occurs with dry mouth, tachycardia and blurred vision?
13. Tremors, muscle rigidity, stooped posture, and shuffling gait oscuras with what disease process
14. What is a state of calm or sleep known as?
16. What is known as having odd or strange tongue and face movements with lip smacking?

Down

3. What is Perphenazine trade name?
5. What is Thioridazine trade name?
8. What consist of severe spasms of the back, tongue and facial muscles with twitching movements?
9. What describes constant pacing with repetitive compulsive movements?
11. What can occur when moving quickly to stand from a sitting position?
12. What disorder can occur with having high fever, confusion, muscle ridgity, and elevated serum CK level and can be deadly?
15. When you are impotence and have a diminished libido this is known as having a

HEART FAILURE MEDICATIONS

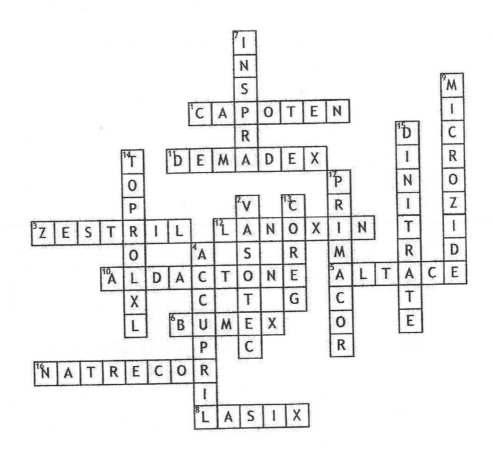

Across

1. What is captopril trade name?
3. What is lisinopril trade name?
5. What is ramipril trade name?
6. What is bumetanide trade name?
8. What is furosemide trade name?
10. What is spironolactone trade name?
11. What is torsemide trade name?
12. What is digoxin trade name?
16. What is nesiritide trade name?

Down

2. What is enalapril trade name?
4. What is quinapril trade name?
7. What is eplerenone trade name?
9. What is Hydrochlorothiazide trade name?
13. What is carvedilol trade name?
14. What is metoprolol Succinate trade name?
15. What is hydralazine with isosorbide trade name?
17. What is inamrinone trade name?

SODIUM, POTASSIUM & CALCIUM CHANNEL BLOCKERS

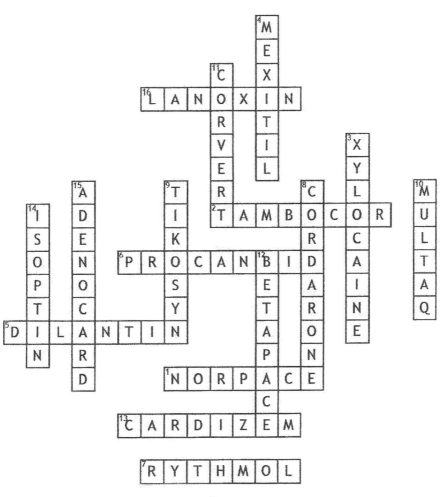

Across

1. What is disopyramide trade name?
2. What is flecainide trade name?
5. What is phenytoin trade name?
6. What is procainamide trade name?
7. What is propafenone trade name?
13. What is diltiazem trade name?
16. What is digoxin trade name?

Down

3. What is lidocaine trade name?
4. What is mexiletine trade name?
8. What is amiodarone trade name?
9. What is dofetilide trade name?
10. What is dronedarone trade name?
11. What is ibutilide trade name?
12. What is sotalol trade name?
14. What is verapamil trade name?
15. What is adenosine trade name?